Gastric Bypass Cookbook

100+ Quick and Easy Recipes for stage 1 and 2 After Gastric Bypass Surgery

Bonus: FREE Report Reveals The Secrets To Lose Weight

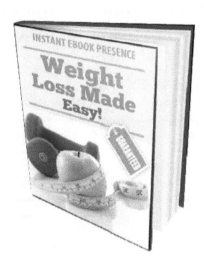

Weight loss doesn't happen from dieting only. Diets are short term solutions to shed extra weight. Diets do not work in the long term because people hate being on a diet (it's ok, you can admit that here). The only long term solution for permanent weight loss is to create new eating habits. This doesn't mean that chocolate will never pass your lips again, but it does mean looking after yourself and watching what you eat...

You can lose weight when you have the right reasons and motivation, and a part of this guide is to help you to find the motivation you need to change your weight...

GO to Get This Guid For FREE
http://www.sportsforsoul.com/weight-loss-2/

Table of Contents

Introduction

Congratulations on downloading your personal copy of *Gastric Bypass Cookbook*. Thank you for doing so.

The following chapters will provide you with many recipes to help you through your gastric bypass diet.

There are plenty of books on this subject on the market, thanks again for choosing this one! Every effort was made to ensure it is full of as much useful information as possible. Please enjoy!

Congratulations on downloading your personal copy of *Gastric Bypass Cookbook*. Thank you for doing so.

Breakfast

Fried Egg on Parmesan Toast

Ingredients

Halved baby tomatoes – optional

Salad leaves – optional

Pepper

Salt

Egg

¼ c parmesan cheese, grated

Instructions

Warm your skillet to a very high heat. Test by dropping some water in the pan, it should sizzle as soon as it hits the pan. It needs to be this hot for this to come out correctly.

Place the cheese in an even layer and spread out so that it is larger than a fried egg. Continue to cook until the cheese starts to bubble up. This shouldn't take but 30 to 50 seconds.

Crack your egg on the cheese. Let the egg cook until the edges have set, this takes about two minutes. Place a lid over the pan and let it continue to cook until the egg has cooked to your liking. The cheese should also be crisped and golden.

Add pepper and salt to your egg. Carefully run a spatula around the cheese and loosen it up. Lift it out and onto a plate.

You can serve with tomatoes and salad leaves if you would like or with your favorite breakfast meats.

Pumpkin Pie Oatmeal

Ingredients

1 scoop vanilla protein powder

¼ c water

Sweetener of choice to taste

2 tbsp oven roasted sliced almonds

¼ c canned pumpkin

Pinch nutmeg

Pinch cinnamon

½ c old fashioned oats

¾ c water

½ c nonfat milk

Instructions

Let some water come up to a boil. Place in nutmeg, cinnamon, and oatmeal. Cook until liquid is gone. Stir occasionally.

When liquid is gone, stir in sweetener, almonds, pumpkin. Set to the side.

Combine protein powder and water in a different bowl. Mix until powder is dissolved, you might have to use a blender.

Pour protein mix over oatmeal and serve.

BBQ Chicken Breakfast Burritos

Ingredients

½ oz 2% sharp cheddar cheese

Dash of salt

1 tbsp barbecue sauce

1 tsp cumin

1 tsp garlic

2 low-fat tortillas

4 oz chicken breast

4 egg whites

Instructions

Scramble the egg whites in a pan sprayed with Pam. Add salt, garlic, and cumin. Stir until the desired doneness. Put half of the chicken breast into a tortilla. Add ½ of the cheese, ½ of the barbecue sauce, and you can add hot sauce if desired. Add half the egg on top. You can add cilantro, onions, and tomatoes if desired. Roll into burritos and serve.

Very Berry Smoothie

Ingredients

½ c nonfat yogurt

½ c nonfat milk

½ c ice

½ c frozen strawberries

½ c frozen blueberries

Instructions

Place all of the above into your blender. Mix until creamy and smooth. Enjoy.

Baked Oatmeal

Ingredients

2 tbsp unsalted slivered almonds

1/3 c craisins

1 tsp vanilla

1 ½ tsp cinnamon

4 tsp Splenda brown sugar

½ c unsweetened applesauce

2 large eggs

1/3 c Splenda

1 c low-fat buttermilk

½ tsp salt

1 ½ tsp baking powder

2 c quick cooking oats

Instructions

Your oven should be at 325. Coat a pie plate with nonstick spray.

Take the dry ingredients and mix them together. Place in the wet and mix well. Place this into your pie plate.

Place in the oven for 40 to 45 minutes. Take out of the oven. Let cool. Cut into 8 equal servings. Store in refrigerator or freezer.

This is the consistency of coffee cake but very good for you. Can be eaten as breakfast, snack, or dessert.

Ricotta Muffins

Ingredients

4 large eggs

2 to 3 tsp Splenda

2 tsp vanilla extract

2 c ricotta cheese

Instructions

Your oven should be at 400. Fill a regular muffin tin with liners. Spray the liners with some nonstick spray.

Stir together all ingredients until smooth. Pour into muffin cups.

Bake 20 to 30 minutes. It will be done when a toothpick inserted comes out clean.

Feel free to add fresh blueberries or blackberries before baking. These freeze great.

Egg Cups

Ingredients

Pepper

Salt

1 tbsp chopped chives

½ c 2% shredded cheddar cheese

6 eggs

6 slices lean deli ham

Instructions

Your oven should be at 350. Coat a six cups in a muffin pan with nonstick spray.

Arrange ham slices to line the muffin cups. The edges might stick up some, that is fine. Bake for 10 minutes. Take out of the oven. Break an egg into each cup. Break the yolks gently. Sprinkle with pepper and salt.

Put back in for another ten minutes. Check the eggs, if they are to your liking remove, sprinkle with chives and cheese. Enjoy.

If they aren't to your liking, continue to cook. Check each minute.

Broccoli Quiche

Ingredients

½ c canned mushrooms

¼ c fat-free half and half

1 large head broccoli

3 oz. low-fat Swiss cheese

¼ c skim milk

1 c egg substitute

Instructions

Your oven should be at 400. A pie plate should be greased with some nonstick spray.

Steam broccoli. Chop.

Add mushrooms and broccoli to pie plate.

Combine half and half, skim milk, and egg substitute. Mix well.

Pour over mushrooms and broccoli. Sprinkle with cheese.

Bake about 40 minutes.

Cut into four equal servings and enjoy.

Breakfast Popsicles

Ingredients

1 cup mixed berries or chopped fruit of choice

½ c oats

½ c 1% milk

1 c Greek yogurt

Instructions

Mix yogurt and milk. Equally, divide mixture into popsicle molds. Put some berries in each. Equally, divide the oatmeal into each mold. Put a wooden stick into each mold and put in the freezer. Freeze a minimum of four hours before eating. If popsicles won't unmold easily. Run under warm water for a few seconds.

PB&J Pancakes

Ingredients

1 c frozen mixed berry blend

4 large egg whites

2 tbsp powdered peanuts

½ c instant oatmeal

½ c low-fat cottage cheese

Instructions

There is a certain order in which these should be placed into the blender. The first ingredient is cottage cheese. The second ingredient should be oatmeal. The third ingredient should be powdered peanuts. The last ingredient will be egg whites. Blend until smooth and pancake batter. Pour into a bowl and add fruit mix. Spray skillet with cooking spray. Makes four to seven pancakes according to size.

Pumpkin Pie Oatmeal

Ingredients

½ c no salt added 1% cottage cheese

1 tsp Truvia

Dash ground ginger

Dash ground cloves

1/8 tsp cinnamon

½ c canned pumpkin

1/3 c old fashioned oats

Instructions

Mix sweetener, spices, pumpkin, and oats in a microwavable bowl. Microwave on high 90 seconds. Stir in cottage cheese. Microwave another 60 seconds. Wait 2 minutes before eating.

Egg Burrito

Ingredients

2 tbsp salsa

1 oz protein of choices like ground beef, chicken, or tofu

1 tbsp shredded Mexican blend cheese

Salt

2 tbsp. plain fat-free Greek yogurt

Pepper

1 egg + 1 egg white

Instructions

Put egg white and egg in small bowl. Beat well. Spray skillet with cooking spray. When hot, pour eggs into heated pan. Spread to coat pan. Let eggs set to allow edges to set. Sprinkle them with pepper and salt. Flip over.

Let the other side cook until completely cooked. Put on a plate. In the center of the egg, add cheese, and protein of choice. Roll up egg to form a burrito. Add Greek yogurt and salsa if desired.

Cottage Cheese Pancakes

Ingredients

3 eggs, lightly beaten

½ tbsp. canola oil

1 c low-fat cottage cheese

½ tsp baking soda

1/3 c all-purpose flour

Instructions

Sift baking soda and flour in small bowl.

Mix rest of the ingredients in large bowl.

Pour flour into wet ingredients and stir to incorporate.

Spray skillet with nonstick spray. Once everything is hot, place 1/3 cup batter in your hot skillet and cook until bubble starts to form on the top. Flip and cook brown another side.

Serve with low-calorie syrup.

Egg Muffin

Ingredients

¼ tsp Italian seasoning

¼ tsp salt

¼ tsp pepper

½ c 1% milk

¾ c shredded low-fat shredded cheese of choice

12 slices turkey bacon

6 large eggs

Instructions

Spray muffin pan with cooking spray. Heat oven to 350.

Put three slices of bacon in bottom of every muffin cup.

Mix all other ingredients together until well mixed. Save ¼ cup shredded cheese. Put ¼ cup of egg mixture in each cup. Sprinkle a bit more cheese over them.

Bake around 25 minutes. The eggs should be set.

Cheese Spiced Pancakes

Ingredients

Pancakes:
Low-fat cooking spray
1 tbsp sugar or artificial sweetener
Pinch salt
½ c AP flour
3 eggs, separated
1 tsp mixed spice, ground
8 oz spreadable goat cheese
Option Adult Toppings:
1 measure brandy
2 oz cranberries
Sweetener

4 tangerines, peeled

Instructions

For making the pancakes, combine the egg yolks, mixed spice, and the cheese. Then beat in the salt and the flour.

Beat the whites of the eggs until they become stiff then whisk in your sweetener of choice. Fold this into the cheese.

If you are making the optional topping, put the sweetener and tangerines in a pan. Stir occasionally until your tangerines start to release their juices and it starts looking a little syrupy. Mix in the brandy and cranberries. Place it to the side until it's time to use it.

Add a bit of cooking spray to your skillet. Let it heat up and add three large spoonfuls of your batter into your pan. Let it cook for two minutes, or the edges form bubbles. Flip the pancake and cook until done. Take out and continue. The batter should make 12 pancakes.

Divide up the pancakes between four different plates spoon the topping over them.

Flour-Less Pancakes

Ingredients

Low-fat spray

Milk to mix

1 banana

1 egg

1 c rolled oats

Instructions

Put the banana, oats, and egg into your food processor and mix it up until it is smooth. Add a bit of milk and blend. Continue adding mix until your mixture reaches a slightly runny consistency. Three tablespoons should be able to help.

Let this mixture sit for around 15 minutes; this will allow the mixture to thicken up a bit.

Spritz some of the cooking spray onto a skillet. Let it heat up and a spoonful of the mixture to make a medallion sized pancake. Place as many on your pan as you can as long as you still have room to flip them. Let the first side cook for a minute and then flip, cooking another minute. Keep the pancakes warm as you finish up your batter.

Serve the pancakes with sugar-free syrup, yogurt, and fruit, or a dust of sugar with a drizzle of lemon. You can also enjoy them plain.

Chocolate Porridge

Ingredients

Sugar-free syrup

Chopped fruits, nuts, or seeds

1 square dark chocolate, unsweetened – optional

1 tbsp cocoa powder

4 tbsp porridge oats

1 c milk, skim

Instructions

Put the chocolate, if using, cocoa powder, oats, and milk into a microwavable bowl.

Heat this in the microwave for two minutes. Mix everything and then cook for another 15 to 20 seconds.

Place in a severing bowl and then add your desired toppings on top.

Ham and Egg Roll Up

Ingredients

20 ham slices

1 c tomatoes, chopped

1 ½ c cheddar cheese, shredded

2 tbsp butter

1 c baby spinach

Pepper

Salt

2 tsp garlic powder

10 eggs

Instructions

Heat up your broiler. Crack the eggs into a bowl and whisk them with the pepper, salt, and garlic powder.

In a skillet, place in the butter and let it melt. Pour in the eggs and scramble them until they are done. Mix in the cheddar, and stir until melted. Fold in the tomatoes and the spinach.

Place two pieces of ham on a cutting board. Add a spoonful of eggs, and then roll it up. Continue until you use up the ham and the eggs.

Put the roll-ups in a baking dish and broil five minutes.

Bunless Breakfast Sandwich

Ingredients

½ avocado, mashed

¼ c cheddar cheese, shredded

2 tbsp water

2 slices bacon, cooked

2 eggs

Instructions

Put two mason jar lids into your skillet and spray the pan with nonstick spray and allow it to heat up. Crack an egg into each of the lids and whisk the egg slightly just to break up the yolks.

Pour some water into the pan and place a lid over the skillet. Let this cook and steam the egg whites. Let this cook for three minutes. Take the lid off and place the cheese on one of the eggs. Let it cook until the cheese has become melty, around a minute.

Place the egg bun that doesn't have the cheese on a plate. Place on the avocado and the bacon. Lay the other egg bun with the cheese side down on top. Enjoy.

Main Dishes

Lamb Souvlaki

Ingredients

16 cherry tomatoes

1 garlic clove, crushed

1 tsp oregano – or ½ tsp dried oregano

2 yellow peppers, cored sliced into bite-sized pieces

12 oz lean lamb, cubed – 12 to 16 pieces

Pepper

1 red onion, sliced into eight wedges

Salt

1 tbsp EVOO

Sauce:

1 tbsp lemon juice

8 oz plain yogurt, low-fat

1 garlic clove, crushed

2 cucumbers, peeled, chopped finely, and drained

Instructions

Stir the pepper, oregano, salt, garlic, and olive oil together. Taste and adjust any of the seasonings that you need to. This is the marinade for your lamb.

Slide the tomatoes, onion, pepper, and lamb onto four different skewers, alternating them, and lay them into a shallow dish. Brush them with the marinade, place a covering over them, and then refrigerate. They should chill for at least two to three hours for the best flavor. When you can, turn them and brush with extra marinade.

You can grill or bake the skewers for five to eight minutes or until the lamb has cooked to medium and are slightly charred. If you want them more well done, cook a little longer.

As they cook, mix together the pepper, garlic, salt, yogurt, lemon juice, and cucumber for your sauce. Serve the sauce along side of the skewers and a slice of pita bread.

Chicken Parmesan

Ingredients

Pepper

Salt

3 tbsp parmesan cheese

½ c hard cheese, low-fat and grated

1 c tomato pasta sauce

1 lb chicken breast fillets, skinless

Instructions

Your oven should be set to 375.

The chicken should be placed in your casserole dish and put the tomato sauce over it.

Add the pepper, salt, parmesan, and the grated hard cheese.

Put this for 25 to 30 minutes in the oven. Make sure the chicken is at 160

This can be served with roasted veggies, pasta, rice, baked potato, or a salad.

Turkey Soup

Ingredients

Salt

Pepper

½ tsp garlic powder

3 cans diced tomatoes

3 tbsp chicken bouillon granules

8 c water

10 oz bag frozen mixed veggies

1 pound ground turkey

1 large zucchini, chopped

2 stalks chopped celery

10 oz mushrooms, sliced

1 large chopped onion

1 tbsp olive oil

Instructions

Sauté zucchini, mushrooms, and onions in pan until soft.

Add ground turkey. Cook until browned.

Put into crockpot. Add remaining ingredients. Place in water. Place on the lid and set on low for six to eight hours.

This recipe freezes well. You may substitute favorite vegetables as you like.

Unstuffed Green Peppers

Ingredients

½ c rice

½ tsp basil

1 tsp garlic powder

1 large diced onion

2 large diced green peppers

2 large diced tomatoes

1 lb lean ground beef

Instructions

Cook half cup rice with 1 cup water per package directions.

Brown ground beef in skillet. Drain. Spoon onto paper towels to drain completely.

Put onion, basil, garlic powder, green peppers, and tomatoes. Let this cook for 15 minutes. Place in cooked rice and ground beef. Stir to combine. Add pepper and salt to taste.

Serve and enjoy.

Italian Chicken

Ingredients

2 lbs skinless, boneless chicken breast

3 c cooked long grain rice

½ c water

1 packet Italian dressing mix

1 can fat-free cream of chicken soup

1 package reduced fat cream cheese

Instructions

Put chicken in your slow cooker.

Combine the water with the dressing mix until well combined. Place this on the chicken.

Place on the lid. Set to low for 8 hours.

Mix the soup and cream cheese together in a bowl.

Set the chicken aside. Shred with two forks.

Pour soup mixture into crock pot and stir to combine.

Put chicken back into crock pot. Stir to combine. Let it continue to cook until everything has heated through.

Serve alongside rice.

Mexican Chicken

Ingredients

¼ c light sour cream

1 ½ tsp taco seasoning

½ can cheddar cheese soup

½ c salsa

1 skinless, boneless chicken breast cut in half

Instructions

Put chicken in slow cooker. Sprinkle taco seasoning over chicken. Stir cheese soup and salsa together and place it over the chicken. Cover. Set for eight hours on low.

Take the chicken out from slow cooker and shred. Put it back in the cooker and mix together. Add sour cream and stir again.

This can be served over rice or used as taco, burrito, or enchilada filling.

Shrimp Ceviche

Ingredients

1 small finely diced red onion

2 serrano chili, seeds and ribs removed, diced

1 bunch cilantro, chopped finely

1 lb medium raw shrimp, peeled and deveined

4 medium tomatoes, diced

1 cup lime juice

Instructions

Combine lime juice and shrimp in a bowl. Place a lid over it and marinate for 15 minutes or until they turn pink. Don't marinate too long. It will make the shrimp tough.

Add cilantro, chili peppers, tomatoes, and onions.

Stir to combine. Season with pepper and salt.

Serve and enjoy.

Chicken Caprese

Ingredients

1 tbsp olive oil

Pepper

1 lb boneless, skinless chicken breast

2 tbsp chopped basil

1 tsp Italian seasoning

3 tbsp balsamic vinegar

4 1 oz slices mozzarella cheese

4 ½-inch slices tomatoes

Instructions

Heat a grill pan or grill.

Place the olive oil on the chicken breasts. Sprinkle with pepper and salt. Sprinkle with Italian seasoning. Grill five minutes each side. Cooking time might vary due to the thickness of chicken.

When chicken is done, place mozzarella cheese on top and cook for another minute.

Remove and place on a plate.

Top with tomato, basil, and pepper.

Drizzle with balsamic vinegar. Serve and enjoy.

Chicken Parmesan

Ingredients

1 tbsp dried

1 tsp garlic powder

¼ c Italian bread crumbs

Crushed red pepper flakes

2 tbsp olive oil

12 oz chicken breast

1 tbsp Parmesan cheese, grated

Instructions

Heat oven to 365.

Filet the chicken breast in two separate pieces. Rub with olive oil.

Mix the above dry ingredients together. Coat each breast piece with dry mixture until well covered.

Bake 20 minutes.

Serve with favorite vegetables or spaghetti.

Salsa Chicken

Ingredients

1 package reduced sodium taco seasoning

½ c reduced fat sour cream

1 can reduced[-fat cream of mushroom soup

1 c salsa

4 skinless, boneless chicken breast

Instructions

Put chicken in slow cooker. Add in the taco seasoning. Place in the salsa. Put on the lid. Cook low for eight hours. Shred chicken. Place chicken back in cooker. Place in sour cream and stir well. Serve with rice.

Taco Stew

Ingredients

1 chopped onion

1 14.5 oz can diced tomatoes

1 15 oz can corn, drained

1 8 oz can tomato sauce

1 10.5 oz can diced tomatoes with chilies

1 15 oz can black beans

1 packet taco seasoning

1 to 2 boneless skinless chicken breast

1 15 oz can kidney beans

Instructions

Add everything to crock pot except chicken. Mix well. Put chicken on top. Place on a lid and cook for eight hours on low. 30 minutes before finished, take out chicken and shred. Put chicken back into cooker and stir.

Ladle into bowls. Serve with sour cream, cheese, sliced green onions, cilantro, or your favorite taco toppings, and tortilla chips.

Mexican Casserole

Ingredients

½ c shredded cheese

4 c water

1 15oz can black beans, drained and rinsed

2 c uncooked brown rice

1 10.75 oz can cheddar cheese soup

1 15.25 oz can sweet corn, undrained

1 diced small onion

1 diced green pepper

1 16 oz jar salsa

2 chicken breasts, boiled and shredded

Instructions

Heat oven to 400.

In large casserole dish, mix brown rice, corn, black beans, soup. Add water and mix thoroughly.

The onion and pepper should be cooked so that they are soft. Place in shredded chicken and heat through. Add this to the rice. Stir to combine well. Cover with lid or foil.

Bake 45 minutes. Stir occasionally. Carefully remove foil. Add a half cup of the cheese. Top with sour cream and tortilla chips.

Chili

Ingredients

2 tsp salt

1 14.5 oz can diced tomatoes

1 medium diced onion

2 14.5 oz cans kidney beans

1 14.5 oz can pureed tomatoes

8 oz chopped mushrooms

2 cloves minced garlic

3 tbsp chili powder

1 tbsp olive oil

1 lb lean ground beef

Instructions

Sauté mushrooms and onion in a pan with olive until soft. Add ground beef; breaking it up. Place in garlic, salt, chili powder, kidney beans, and tomatoes. Stir well to combine. Let it come to a boil. Turn to a simmer for about two hours.

Serve over rice with sour cream, shredded cheese, and avocado as toppings.

Pepper Steak

Ingredients

1 14.5 oz can diced tomatoes

1 can mushrooms

1 to 2 red bell peppers

1 medium chopped onions

¼ c salsa

1.5 to 2 lbs lean round steak, sliced into strips

Instructions

Put the above in your slow cooker. Place on the lid. Place on low. Cook 8 hours.

Serve with mashed potatoes or rice.

Sante Fe Soup

Ingredients

2 c water

2 11 oz. cans shoepeg corn, drained

1 large chopped onion

1 15 oz can kidney beans, undrained

2 14 oz. cans diced tomatoes, undrained

1 15 oz can pinto beans, undrained

1 envelope ranch dressing mix

1 10 oz. can tomatoes with green chilies, undrained

1 15 oz can black beans, undrained

2 envelopes taco seasoning

1 lb chicken breast, boiled and chopped

Instructions

Place the above in your slow cooker. Give a good stir. Cover.
Set to low. Cook for four hours.

Beef and Gravy

Ingredients

½ tsp garlic powder

1 can 98% fat-free cream of mushroom soup

1 stalk diced celery

1 medium sliced onion

2 tbsp flour

1 lb stew beef

½ tsp pepper

Instructions

Place onion across the bottom of crock pot. Mix garlic, flour, and pepper in a bowl. Cover the meat with mixture. Put meat on top of onions. Pour soup over meat. Top with diced celery. Cover. Set to low. Cook eight hours.

Serve over rice or mashed potatoes.

Rainbow Trout

Ingredients

2 tsp olive oil

Pinch salt

¼ tsp pepper

¼ tsp celery seeds

1 1/3 tbsp chopped parsley

3 tbsp yellow cornmeal

8 oz. rainbow trout fillets

Instructions

Clean and rinse fish. Check for bones. Pat dry.

Mix parsley, celery seed, pepper, salt, and cornmeal.

Coat fish with mixture. Press to make sure it sticks.

Put olive oil in skillet. Cook a few minutes on each side. Fish will be brown and crispy. Should flake easily when pierced with a fork.

Creamy Spinach and Chicken Bake

Ingredients

1 c shredded Mozzarella

2 tsp garlic powder

¼ c Parmesan cheese

½ c fat-free sour cream

10 oz baby spinach

2 c diced cooked chicken breast

½ c light mayonnaise

Instructions

Your oven should be at 350. Coat a casserole dish with nonstick spray. Steam spinach, drain well. Mix garlic powder, cheese, mayonnaise, and sour cream. Pour half into casserole dish. Add chicken and spinach. Cover with remaining sour cream mixture. Bake 45 minutes until heated and bubbly.

Broiled Parmesan Tilapia

Ingredients

Salt

1 tsp chopped garlic

4 4 oz. tilapia filet

1 tbsp. lime juice

2 tbsp. grated parmesan cheese

½ tsp dried dill

1 tbsp light mayonnaise

Instructions

Heat oven to broil.

Put tilapia on broiling pan and sprinkle with salt and half of the dill. Put on the top rack and broil for three minutes. While broiling, mix the remaining ingredients. Don't forget the remaining dill. Take tilapia out of the oven, spread parmesan mixture over filets. Place in oven for three more minutes.

Creole Shrimp

Ingredients

4 c cook rice

1 ½ lbs peeled and deveined shrimp

6 c fat-free chicken broth

½ tsp thyme

½ tsp oregano

½ tsp red pepper flakes

6 tbsp tomato paste

2 medium chopped green bell pepper

4 chopped celery ribs

3 cloves minced garlic

2 medium chopped onions

2 tbsp olive oil

Instructions

Heat a pot with some oil. Place in garlic and all vegetables. Cook until soft. Place in thyme, red pepper flakes, oregano, and tomato paste. Cook until fragrant. Add broth and allow it to come to a boil. Cook until beginning to thicken around 30 minutes. Add shrimp and cook until opaque.

Serve over cooked rice.

Sweet Potato and Chicken Stew

Ingredients

Dash of oregano

Pinch of cumin

2 c 99% fat-free chicken broth

1 medium diced onion

1 ½ cups frozen corn

2 c fat-free salsa

1 large diced sweet potato

12 oz boneless skinless chicken breast, diced

Instructions

Put the above, except corn, into slow cooker. Cover. Set to low. Cook six hours. 30 minutes before done, add corn. Cook remaining 30 minutes.

Cola Chicken

Ingredients

1 c ketchup

3 boneless skinless chicken breast

1 12 oz can diet cola of choice

Instructions

Sear the chicken first in your pan. Pour cola and ketchup on top. Bring to boil. Cover. Simmer about 45 minutes. Uncover, bring back to a boil and boil until it thickens up and sticks to chicken. Watch the chicken carefully during this stage as it will burn.

Cranberry Chicken

Ingredients

Salt

Pepper

6 tsp Splenda

1 c fresh cranberries

2 5 oz chicken breast

Instructions

Put water, Splenda, and cranberries in a pot. Let it come to a boil. Cook until cranberries pop. Refrigerate overnight. Put cranberries in a crock pot. Add chicken, pepper, and salt. Cover. Set to low. Cook for five hours.

Sticky Chicken

Ingredients

½ tsp black pepper

1 tsp cayenne pepper

½ tsp garlic powder

1 c chopped onion

1 tsp salt

3 to 4 lb roasting chicken

1 tsp onion powder

1 tsp thyme

2 tsp paprika

1 tsp white pepper

Instructions

Put the above spices in small bowl and mix thoroughly. Clean out the chicken. Pat dry. Rub spice mixture on chicken. Don't forget the inside. Put in resealable bag, and let sit in fridge overnight

When ready to bake chicken, let it come to room temp. Heat oven to 275. Place onions in the cavity of the chicken. Place in baking pan. Bake uncovered for five hours. The juices will start to caramelize, and chicken will brown up. Ignore the chicken's pop up thermometer if it has one. When done, take and let it red before you crave it.

Italian Chicken Breasts

Ingredients

Salt

1 c chicken broth

3 c sliced mushrooms

½ tsp pepper blend

4 boneless, skinless chicken breasts

1 tsp Italian seasoning

1 tsp paprika

Instructions

Mix all spices together. Rub this over the chicken. Add chicken to warmed skillet. Cook until browned. Turn and brown another side. Reduce heat. Mix in the broth and mushrooms. Place on lid and let cook for 20 minutes or the chicken reaches 160.

White Chicken Chili

Ingredients

¼ tsp cayenne pepper

2 tsp ground cumin

1 c salsa

2 diced chili peppers

2 seeded, diced jalapenos

1 tbsp olive oil

2 medium chopped onions

1 lb great northern beans (soaked overnight in water)

2 cloves minced garlic

6 cups diced cooked chicken breasts

1 ½ tsp oregano

Instructions

Simmer the beans with half the garlic and onions in chicken broth for two hours. Be sure the beans are soft. Add salsa and chicken.

In olive oil sauté onions, spices, and peppers. Add to bean mixture. Simmer an additional hour.

Serve with reduced fat cheese or light sour cream.

Brown Sugar Garlic Chicken

Ingredients

2 tbsp butter

Black pepper

4 tsp brown sugar

1 clove garlic

12 oz boneless, skinless chicken breast

Instructions

Place butter in a pan and melt. Place in garlic, and cook until it smells. Place in chicken breasts and cook through. Sprinkle with pepper.

When chicken is cooked through, add brown sugar to the top. Allow to melt. This should take about five minutes.

Serve with favorite vegetable. It is great on top of a salad.

Black Bean Soup

Ingredients

2 c chicken broth

1 cup salsa

2 cans black beans, washed and drained

Instructions

Add all ingredients to pot and heat through. Use an immersion blender or put in blender to make it a creamy black bean soup.

Garnish with fresh cilantro or herbs of choice.

Mushrooms and Beef

Ingredients

1 can low-fat cream of mushroom soup

½ cup water

1 lb lean stew meat

8 oz sliced mushrooms

1 packet onion soup mix

Instructions

Brown meat in skillet. Put meat in slow cooker. Place in mushrooms. Mix water, soup mix, and soup. Pour over beef and mushrooms. Cover. Set to low. Cook for eight hours.

Serve over rice or noodles.

Parmesan Tilapia

Ingredients

Pepper

1 tsp garlic powder, divided

4 sprigs fresh dill

¼ c grated parmesan

2 tsp non-fat plain yogurt

2 tsp light mayonnaise

2 tilapia fillets

Instructions

Heat oven to broil.

If filets are frozen, thaw completely. Put cheese, yogurt, and mayonnaise in a bowl. Mix well.

Put aluminum foil on cookie sheet. Spray with cooking spray.

Put tilapia fillets on cookie sheet 2-inches apart. Spread cheese mixture over each filet. Separate dill with hands and sprinkle over fish. Sprinkle with garlic powder and black pepper. Put the cookie sheet in oven about 6 inches below broiler.

Watch this carefully. It will take about five to seven minutes to cook completely. When cheese starts browning, check every 30 seconds. Fish is going to flake easily when cooked fully.

Turn off broiler and leave fish in the oven. Wait five minutes.

Take out of the oven and serve with a favorite side.

Low-fat Cheeseburger Pie

Ingredients

¾ c shredded cheddar cheese

4 tomato slices

1 clove chopped garlic

½ c chopped onion

¾ cup heart smart Bisquick

¼ c water

1 tbsp Worcestershire sauce

1 c fat-free cottage cheese

1 lb ground turkey

1 egg

Instructions

Heat oven to 350.

Brown turkey in skillet. Add garlic and onions.

While cooking, combine water and baking mix until well combined. Roll dough flat to cover pie plate. Place dough in pie plate.

Add Worcestershire to meat.

In additional bowl mix egg and cottage cheese.

Pour turkey mixture into a pie plate. Top with cottage cheese mixture. Top with cheese.

Add on tomatoes. Cook for about 30 to 40 minutes.

Diet Cola Sloppy Joes

Ingredients

2 tbsp white vinegar

1 tbsp Worcestershire sauce

Garlic powder

2 tsp dry mustard

2/3 c reduced sugar ketchup

1 c diet cola

1 lb 96% lean ground beef

Instructions

Brown beef in skillet. Drain. Put beef back in skillet. Place all the rest in and mix well. Cook 15 minutes or until it thickens.

Serve on buns.

Quick Chili

Ingredients

1 tbsp chili powder

½ c salsa

1 tbsp cumin powder

1 15 oz can kidney beans, rinsed and drained

1 28 oz can stewed tomatoes

1 15 oz can pinto beans, rinsed and drained

½ c chopped onion

1 lb ground turkey

Instructions

Brown the turkey with onion. Add salsa, cumin, chili powder, garlic, tomatoes, and beans. Cook until heated through.

Serve with baked potato, cooked rice, cooked pasta, or cornbread. Top with cheese.

Applesauce Peanut Chicken

Ingredients

1 15 oz jar unsweetened applesauce

Salt

Pepper

½ c powdered peanuts

1/8 c Splenda brown sugar

¼ cup yellow mustard

2 ½ lbs chicken pieces

Instructions

Sauté chicken in pan until almost done. Add applesauce, powdered peanuts, brown sugar, and mustard. Stir together. Simmer until chicken temp reaches 165.

Chicken Chili

Ingredients

½ tsp black pepper

3 c water

2 c pinto beans that have soaked overnight in water.

1 tsp salt

1 tbsp chili powder

3 ¼ cups salsa Verde or green enchilada sauce

1 ½ tsp ground cumin

2 cans chopped green chilies

1 ½ c cooked chopped chicken

1 medium chopped onion

Instructions

Sauté chicken and onion with spices until onion is soft. Add beans, water, enchilada sauce, and chilies.

Simmer until beans are tender.

This is good topped with cheese and tortilla chips.

Creamy Chicken

Ingredients

¼ c Italian dressing

1 clove chopped garlic

½ c low sodium chicken broth

1 small chopped onion

1 can low-fat cream of chicken soup

8 oz. low-fat cream cheese

3 lbs boneless, skinless chicken breast

Instructions

Spray slow cooker with nonstick spray.

Put the chicken inside and drizzle with dressing.

Sauté garlic and onions in a pan with cooking spray until soft. Add cream cheese, broth, and soup. Combine until creamy. Add to slow cooker.

Place on lid, set to six hours on low.

Serve with vegetables of choice. Add the vegetables to the crock pot for a one pot meal.

Mexican Chicken Stew

Ingredients

1 can black beans, undrained

1 can chopped green chilies

1 can black olives

1 can Mexican style chili beans, undrained

1 can diced tomatoes

1 pkg taco seasoning

2 to 3 chicken breasts

Instructions

Put chicken in crock pot. Add diced tomatoes, black beans, chili beans, taco seasoning, black olives, chopped green chilies. Don't stir. Cover. Set to low. Cook for eight hours.

Remove the chicken and shred it up. Place it back into the cooker. Mix well. Serve eight on a tortilla or with tortilla chips. Top with shredded cheese, tomatoes, and chopped lettuce.

Stuffed Peppers

Ingredients

1 ½ lbs lean ground beef

1 tsp garlic powder

1 cup chopped onion

1 ½ cups minute rice, brown

1 large egg

1 tsp salt

2 cups tomato sauce

1 tsp black pepper

4 bell peppers

Instructions

Slice all of the peppers in half. Take out the ribs and seeds.

Combine remaining ingredients except for a cup of the tomato sauce and bell peppers.

Split this between the bell peppers

Spread a half cup of the tomato sauce in the slow cooker. Place in the peppers. Top with the rest of the sauce

Place on the lid. Set to low. Cook six hours.

Pork Chops

Ingredients

Salt

Pepper

½ c water

2 tbsp corn starch

1 ½ c chicken broth

2 tbsp olive oil

½ c thin sliced onion

½ c each yellow, red, green bell peppers, sliced thin

4 3 oz pork chops

Instructions

Sauté pork in olive oil until browned. Take out of the pan. Set to the side.

Toss in the pepper and onion in the pan and sauté until they are caramelized and aromatic. Pour in the broth and put the pork back in.

Pork should cook until no longer pink, so about 15 minutes. Remove from pan.

Stir corn starch into cold water until dissolved. Place in the pan and let thicken.

Add pepper and salt to taste.

White Chicken Chili

Ingredients

Parsley flakes
1 red bell pepper, diced and seeded
Onion powder
2 cans low sodium chicken broth
½ diced sweet onion
Garlic powder
Cumin
1 tbsp olive oil
1 to 2 tbsp canned green chilies, drained
1 lb boneless, skinless chicken breast, cubed
1 cup chunky salsa
1 heaping tsp minced garlic

3 cans great northern beans

Instructions

Heat Dutch oven and add olive oil. Mix the onion, garlic, and bell pepper into the pot, and they should cook until soft

Add chicken. Sprinkle with cumin, onion powder, and garlic powder. Brown up until no longer pink

Place in chilies, salsa, chicken broth, and beans. Stir well.

Add ¼ tsp parsley flakes, ½ tsp onion powder, ½ tsp garlic powder, and 1 ½ tsp cumin.

Heat until simmering. Simmer 20 minutes.

If you want it thicker, you can use a slurry of ¼ cup warm water and 3 tbsp corn starch mixed together before adding to pan. Let this simmer a couple more minutes until to desired thickness.

Leftovers freeze extremely well.

Chicken and Artichoke Casserole

Ingredients

1 can reduced-fat cream of mushroom soup

1 14 oz can artichoke hearts, packed in brine, drained

2 lbs. boneless, skinless chicken breast

Instructions

Cut chicken into 2-inch pieces and add to crock pot. Cut artichoke hearts in half. Add to crock pot. Add soup. Cover. Set to low. Cook five hours. Stir to combine. Serve and enjoy.

Baked Chicken and Veggies

Ingredients

Pepper

1 tsp thyme

½ c water

1 chicken, skin removed, cut into pieces

1 quartered large onion

6 sliced carrots

4 sliced potatoes

Instructions

Heat oven to 400. Put onions, carrots, and potatoes in roasting pan. Place chicken on top. Mix pepper, thyme, and water. Pour over vegetables and chicken. Bake at least an hour until tender and browned. Internal temperature should be 165. Baste chicken with juices during cooking.

Black Bean and Pork Verde Stew

Ingredients

1 tsp red pepper flakes

1 14.5 oz can no salt added black beans, washed and drained

2 canned chipotle pepper in adobo sauce, minced

3 garlic cloves

1 tsp ground cumin

1 packet taco seasoning

1 14 oz can no salt added chicken broth

1 ¼ c chopped onions

1 lb pork loin, trimmed and cubed

1 tsp adobo sauce

1 14.5 oz can no salt added diced tomatoes in juice

2 tsp olive oil

Instructions

Heat up a Dutch oven with oil. Place in pork. Cook until browned. Place in garlic and onion cook until softened. Add seasoning packet, cumin, chipotle peppers, and sauce. Stir to mix. Add beans, tomatoes, red pepper flakes, and broth. Stir. Let it come to boil. Let it cook lightly. Cover with a lid and cook for another 40 to 45 minutes or until the pork is tender. Serve in bowls over rice.

Asian Lettuce Wraps

Ingredients

1 small cucumber, seeded and sliced into 1-inch strips
8 small butter lettuce leaves
3 tbsp sherry cooking wine
1 8 oz. can water chestnuts, drained and minced
¼ tsp salt
½ lb ground chicken breast
1 green onion, chopped
1 tsp toasted sesame oil
2 tbsp. hoisin sauce
1 c minced onion
2 packets sugar substitute
1 tbsp unsalted peanut butter
1 tsp minced ginger
2 tsp hot pepper sauce
2 tsp low sodium soy sauce
1 tbsp minced garlic

1 8 oz can bamboo shoots, drained and minced

Instructions

Combine sugar substitute, hot sauce, soy sauce, peanut butter, hoisin sauce, sherry, water chestnuts, and bamboo shoots. Mix well. Set to the side.

Spray skillet with cooking spray. Warm and add in the onion cooking until it turns soft. Stir in garlic, cooking until it smells. Turn up the heat. Add salt, ginger, and ground chicken. Breaking up chicken so that it cooks all the way through. Add bamboo shoot mixture. Heat through. Stir in sesame oil. Take off heat.

Divide chicken equally onto the lettuce leaves. Top with green onion and cucumber. Serve and enjoy.

Black Bean and Turkey Sloppy Joes

Ingredients

1 tsp Mrs. Dash onion and herb blend

1 14.5 oz can diced tomatoes with green chilies

1 ½ c low sodium tomato juice

1 tbsp. olive oil

1 tsp paprika

2 tsp chili powder

1 medium chopped onion

1 tsp minced garlic

1 6 oz can tomato paste

1 14.5 oz can black beans, drained and rinsed

1 lb ground turkey

Instructions

Brown turkey up, and drain the fat off. Place in all of the other ingredients and cook until as thick as you want it.

Serve on buns or bread.

Taco Chicken

Ingredients

¼ c nonfat sour cream

1 c salsa

4 4 oz. chicken breast

1 pkg taco seasoning

Instructions

Heat oven to 375.

Place taco seasoning and chicken in resealable bag. Shake to coat. Place in greased casserole. Bake 30 minutes. Coat the top with salsa five minutes before it's done. Top with sour cream just before serving.

Fajita Chicken

Ingredients

Garlic powder

1 bag frozen pepper and onion blend

3 c chunky salsa

1 packet taco seasoning

3 lb. frozen boneless chicken breast

Instructions

Put frozen chicken breasts in crock pot. Sprinkle with taco seasonings. Spoon some salsa over each one. Sprinkle with garlic powder. Dump frozen peppers and onions on top.

Place on lid and set to eight hours on low.

Serve as is or shred for tacos, fajitas, nachos, taco salad, burritos, or to top a baked potato. You will have leftovers.

Chicken and Vegetables

Ingredients

1 8oz can tomato sauce

3 to 4 cloves minced garlic

3 16 oz cans diced tomatoes

3 lb bag boneless skinless chicken breast

8 oz sliced mushrooms

3 small slice zucchini

4 yellow or red sliced bell peppers

2 small diced Vidalia onions

Instructions

Cube chicken. Place in large pan with garlic and onion. Cook. Season to taste.

Continue to cook unto almost done. Add tomato sauce, canned tomatoes, mushrooms, zucchini, and bell peppers. Place a lid on it and let it cook about 20 minutes. Veggies should be tender.

Serve as is or over rice. Any leftovers freeze well.

Spicy Peanut Vegetarian Chili

Ingredients

1 16 oz can white beans, washed and drained

2 cups vegetable broth

1 c chopped onion

2/3 c powdered peanuts

2 cloves minced garlic

1 28 oz. can diced tomatoes

1 tbsp. peanut oil

1 tsp chipotle chili powder

1 16 oz. can black beans, washed and drained

¼ tsp dried oregano

1 15 oz. can tomato sauce

2 tbsp. chili powder

Instructions

Heat up a Dutch oven with some oil. Place the garlic and onion in and allow them to cook until they turn tender. Stir in salt, oregano, pepper, and chili powder. Cook until fragrant. Add broth, tomato sauce, tomatoes, powdered peanuts, corn, and beans. Let boil. Simmer about 30 minutes.

Halloumi Wraps

Ingredients

Dressing:

1 tsp olive oil

2 tbsp sweet chili sauce

Filing and Salad:

4 wraps, low-carb

6 radishes, sliced

1 lime, juiced

4 spring onions, sliced

2 celery stalks, sliced

1 head lettuce, leaves separated

9 oz. Halloumi cheese

Instructions

Stir all of the dressing parts together.

Slice the halloumi into eight slices and coat them with the dressing.

Place them on a grill or in a pan and brown on both sides for three minutes. They should become brown and crisp on the outside.

While they cook, combine the radishes, spring onions, celery, and lettuce together. Add all the rest of the dressing on your salad and toss everything together.

Split this salad between all of your wraps and place two of the grilled cheese slices on each of them. Serve this immediately.

Sichuan Roasted Eggplant

Ingredients

6 spring onions, chopped – garnish
Drizzle sesame oil – optional
1 tbsp dark soy sauce
3 eggplants
Pepper
2 tbsp olive oil
Salt
2 tsp honey
2 tbsp sweet chili sauce
1 red chili, chopped finely
3 tsp ginger, chopped
2 tbsp tomato paste

4 garlic cloves, crushed

Instructions

You should have your oven at 400. Place foil or a silicone baking sheet onto a cookie sheet, so that clean up is easy.

Combine the pepper, honey, salt, sweet chili sauce, oil, soy sauce, tomato paste, chili, and ginger together.

Slice the eggplants in half lengthwise then make a deep score, crisscross marks into the eggplants. Make sure the skins don't get cut. Put the eggplants on your baking sheet and spoon the paste that you created earlier over all of the halves. Loosely cover eggplants with foil and let them cook for 30 minutes.

Take the foil off of them and let it continue to cook for another 30 minutes. It should be tender and brown. Drizzle the top with some sesame oil if you want to, and let them stand for five minutes.

Top with a scattering of onions.

Vegetable Stir-Fry

Ingredients

Small handful of cilantro – optional

4 tbsp soy sauce

2 red peppers, sliced and cored

11 oz baby corn, halved

2 garlic cloves, crushed

1 lb Chinese leaf lettuce, shredded

1 lb oriental mushrooms

1 onion, sliced

1 chili, chopped finely

2 tsp sesame oil

Instructions

Oil a wok and heat it up over medium heat.

Place the garlic and the chili and let them cook for 30 seconds.

Place in the peppers, corn, Chinese lettuce, and mushrooms. Stir-fry this mixture for about four minutes, or until they become tender-crisp.

Pour the soy sauce over everything and toss it together.

Serve with cilantro.

Lemon Chicken Kebabs

Ingredients

2 tsp basil – garnish

1 tbsp lemon zest

Skewer vegetables – like zucchini and tomatoes

4 chicken breasts, cubed

2 lemons, juice

2 tbsp olive oil

Dipping Sauce:

3 tbsp chopped basil

2 garlic cloves, crushed

8 oz plain goat's cheese yogurt

½ lemon, juice, and zest

Instructions

In a bowl, mix the lemon juice, salt, lemon zest, pepper, and oil. Put the chicken and coat it in the sauce. Place a covering over the bowl and let it marinate in the fridge for around 30 minutes.

While that marinates, combine the pepper, lemon juice, basil, salt, lemon zest, garlic, and yogurt to make the dipping sauce. Place this in the fridge until ready to be used.

Thread the veggies and chicken onto eight to 12 skewers, alternating them. Grill the kebabs for five to eight minutes on every side, making sure to turn them often. Baste them as they cook with the leftover marinade

Once the chicken is done, serve them with the dipping sauce and top with some basil.

Veggie Chilli

Ingredients

Sprigs cilantro – optional garnish

1 tsp chopped rosemary

1 red onion, sliced

½ c strong grated cheese, low-fat

2 tsp chipotle paste

12 oz cherry tomato and basil sauce

14 oz. black beans, washed and drained

7 oz. Romano peppers, sliced and seeded

Nonstick spray, low-fat

Instructions

Coat a skillet with a generous amount of the nonstick spray. Let it heat up and add the rosemary, red onion, and peppers. Let this cook for five minutes.

Place in the chipotle paste, cherry tomato and basil sauce, and beans. Let this mixture simmer for around ten minutes. The peppers should become tender.

Serve the chili with cilantro and grated cheese.

Lamb Koftas

Ingredients

2 tbsp dressing, fat-free
2 tbsp mint, chopped
4 oz feta cheese, light
8 oz cherry tomatoes, halved
½ cucumber, sliced and halved
2 tbsp parsley, chopped
1 ½ oz. craisins
½ tsp ground coriander
½ tsp cumin
1 garlic clove, crushed
½ small onion, chopped
8 oz lean ground lamb

2 oz bulgur wheat

Instructions

Place the wheat into a skillet. Place in water to cover it and let it come up to a boil. Cook five minutes. The wheat should become tender, and drain off the water.

Combine the garlic, onion, wheat, and lamb together. Mix in the parsley, craisins, coriander, and cumin. Mix until everything comes together. Split the meat up into 12 portions.

Heat up your broiler or a grill. Take one of the 12 portions and press around a skewer, tightly, to make an oval. Continue this with the rest of the portions. Put this on a broiler pan or on the grill, and cook for around ten minutes. Make sure you turn them so that they are cooked through and browned on both sides.

Meanwhile, combine the rest of the parsley, mint, feta, tomatoes, and cucumbers and toss them in the dressing. Serve with the koftas.

Beef and Broccoli Stir-Fry

Ingredients

4 scallions, shredded

1 tsp rice vinegar

4 tbsp oyster sauce

2 red chilies, sliced thinly

5 oz shiitake mushrooms, sliced

8 oz broccoli, cut in half

1 red onion, sliced thickly

Low-fat spray

12 oz beef steak, cut into ½ inch strips

1 tsp ginger, grated

1 tbsp light soy sauce

Instructions

Combine the steak, ginger, and soy sauce and allow the steak to sit for 15 minutes.

Spray a wok with low-fat spray. Let it heat up and place in the steak mixture. For four to five minutes, stir-fry the steak until browned and cooked. Place the steak in a clean bowl for later.

Place the chili, mushrooms, broccoli, and onion in the wok and let it cook for five minutes, or until all the veggies have become tender. Add a little water or more low-fat spray when needed to make sure that it doesn't burn.

Place the steak and its juices back to the wok and mix in the rice vinegar and oyster sauce. Cook for another couple of minutes until everything is good and heated through.

Garnish with a scattering of scallions.

Thai Sea Bass

Ingredients

1 tbsp soy sauce

2 tbsp chopped cilantro – optional

2 sea bass fillets

2 garlic cloves, crushed

3 tbsp. oil

4 tsp ginger, grated

1 lemon, juice and zest

1 mild red chili, sliced and seeded

2 spring onions, chopped

8 oz. bok choy, quartered

1 tbsp. fish sauce

4 oz. asparagus, trimmed

Instructions

Your oven should be at 400.

Put the onions, bok choy, and asparagus into a roasting pan.

Mix together the lemon juice, lemon zest, fish sauce, oil, ginger, soy sauce, chili, and garlic together. Pour the mixture over the vegetables and toss to coat. Then, place the veggies in the oven and allow it to cook for five minutes.

Take them out and set the sea bass on top. Place this for another eight minutes in the oven, or until your sea bass is cooked all the way through. It should flake easily with poked with a fork, and it should be opaque.

Place the rest of the dressing over the fish, top with cilantro, and enjoy.

Mini Meatloaves

Ingredients

Toppings: dill pickle, mustard, or ketchup – these are optional

¾ c shredded cheese, reduced-fat

¼ tsp pepper

1 tsp onion powder

1 lb. ground beef, extra lean

2 tsp mustard

1 c onion, chopped

½ tsp salt

1 tsp garlic powder

3 tbsp. ketchup

¼ c egg whites

¼ c panko breadcrumbs, whole wheat

½ c green bell pepper, chopped

Instructions

Your oven should be set at 375. Coat a regular cupcake tin with cooking spray.

Mix together all of the above, except for the cheese. Make sure it is well combined. Distribute the meat into between the cup and smooth across the tops.

Bake them for 35 minutes or until the edges have browned up and it is firm.

Grate some cheese and sprinkle it on top and return it to the oven for another three minutes to melt the cheese.

Serve with the desired toppings.

Stuffed Chicken

Ingredients

Pepper
Salt
Tomato sauce
Mozzarella cheese
½ c ricotta cheese
½ pack of frozen spinach, squeezed
1 egg
¼ c parmesan, divided
½ c breadcrumbs

4 chicken cutlets, pounded thin

Instructions

Combine half of the parmesan with the breadcrumbs and place on the side.

Mix the remaining parmesan, spinach, and ricotta together in a bowl. You should make sure that the spinach has been completely squeezed dry.

Place the cutlets onto a cutting board spread two tablespoons of the spinach mixture over the top.

Roll the cutlets up and secure with toothpicks.

In a shallow dish beat up the eggs.

Coat cutlets in egg and then the breadcrumbs.

Put the cutlets seam side down into a casserole dish that is coated with nonstick spray. Your oven should be at 425. Bake 25 minutes.

Take the casserole dish out and top with tomato sauce and mozzarella.

Cook for another five minutes and enjoy.

Chicken Nuggets

Ingredients

Nonstick spray

2 tbsp parmesan

3 tbsp. panko breadcrumbs

¼ tsp pepper

¼ tsp oregano

½ tsp garlic salt

½ tsp Italian herbs

½ tsp salt

3 tsp canola oil

1 lb chicken breasts, diced

Instructions

Your oven should be at 450.

Toss the chicken with the oil. Sprinkle with the pepper, oregano, garlic salt, Italian herbs, and salt. Massage all of the spices into you chicken.

Place the parmesan cheese, panko, and the chicken into a bag and seal the bag closed. Shake the bag and squeeze the chicken a few times to get it coated well.

Grease up a cookie sheet with baking spray.

Place the chicken nuggets on the cookie sheet in one layer.

Spritz the top of the chicken with more baking spray.

Cook it for about eight minutes or until t

Let it cook for eight minutes, or until it is no longer pink.

Crustless Pizza Bites

Ingredients

Pizza toppings of your choice

Pizza sauce

Mozzarella cheese, shredded

Thick cut Canadian bacon

Instructions

First, you need to grease up your regular muffin tin. Place three Canadian bacon slices like a three leaf clover over the cups. Press down gently to press them into the cups. They don't like to stay that will, but it will be okay. Once you add the toppings, it will settle better.

Gather together your cheese, sauce, and toppings.

Place a tablespoon of the pizza sauce into each of the pizza cups.

Add in as many pizza toppings as you want, and as your cups can hold.

Sprinkle over with a good amount of the mozzarella cheese.

Your oven should be at 350. Place the pizza inside and bake it for 27 minutes or until things start to golden and it becomes bubbly. Make sure not to burn the pizza.

Pop the pizzas out with a fork. A small amount of juice may be in the bottom of the cup, just discard that. Enjoy the pizzas either with a fork or by hand.

Mini Chicken Parmesan

Ingredients

¾ c mozzarella cheese, reduced-fat
¾ c pasta sauce
2 cloves garlic, minced
¾ c parmesan cheese
1/3 tsp pepper
¾ tsp dried thyme
¾ tsp salt
½ small onion, chopped
¾ tsp oregano
¾ tsp dried basil
6 tbsp breadcrumbs
1 egg white
1 egg

1 ½ lb ground chicken breast

Instructions

Your oven should be at 350. Lightly coat a regular muffin tin with some non-stick spray.

Mix together the parmesan, pepper, onion, salt, garlic, oregano, thyme, basil, breadcrumbs, egg whites, egg, and chicken. Do not overmix. Fold the mixture just until you see everything is well incorporated and is distributed throughout the chicken.

Place the mixture evenly between the 12 cups. Place the pasta sauce over the muffins. Place this in your oven and cook 20 minutes. Take it out of the oven and add around a tablespoon of shredded cheese and place it back in the oven for another two minutes making sure the cheese melt on top. Pop them out with a knife or fork and enjoy.

Desserts

Coconut Pistachio Fingers

Ingredients

Extra pistachios

¼ c coconut flakes, unsweetened

2 tbsp olive oil

4 tbsp sugar-free syrup – or maple or agave syrup

Pinch salt

1 c rolled oats

1 c shelled pistachio

Instructions

Your oven should be set at 350. Place greased foil or parchment paper in an eight-inch square dish.

Put the salt, pistachios, and oats in your food processor and pulse them up until they are very fine.

Turn on the processor, and while it's running, add in the oil and syrup until it starts to form a crumbly but moist dough. It shouldn't stick together yet.

Place this in the dish and press it down with a spoon until level. Sprinkle the extra pistachios and the coconut flakes on top.

Bake this for 12 minutes. It should be cooked through and golden. Lift the cookies out by lifting up the foil or parchment. Let it cool on a rack.

Cut it into 16 long cookies and keep it stored in a container.

Peanut Butter Muffins

Ingredients

4 tbsp protein powder

½ c mini chocolate chips

½ tsp salt

1 tbsp vanilla

¼ c honey

2 eggs

1 c creamy peanut

1 tsp baking powder

2 bananas, extremely ripe

Instructions

Your oven should be at 400.

Place the above, except chocolate chips, into your blender. Mix everything up for around 30 seconds, or until it is well mixed.

Place in a bowl and lightly mix in the chocolate chips.

Spray a regular muffin tin with nonstick spray and add batter into each cup.

Cook these for 12 to 14 minutes, or until they have set.

PB Mug Cake

Ingredients

1 tbsp chopped peanuts

1/8 tsp vanilla

1 tbsp powdered peanut butter

1 tbsp vanilla soymilk, light

2 tbsp egg whites

½ packet of sweetener

¼ tsp baking powder

1 tbsp vanilla protein powder

1 tbsp coconut flour

Instructions

Coat a mug with cooking spray. Place in the sweetener, baking powder, powdered peanut butter, protein powder, and flour. Combine everything together.

Mix in two tablespoons of water, vanilla extract, soymilk, and egg whites.

Place in the microwave for a minute and 15 seconds, or until it has set up.

Slide a knife around the cake. Set a plate over the cup and quickly flip it. Shake the cake free from the cup. Top with some extra peanuts.

Salted Caramel Cheesecakes

Ingredients

Crust:
2/3 c lightly sweetened fiber cereal
2 tbsp Greek yogurt cream cheese, low-fat and softened
Filling:
½ c sweetener
1/3 c whey protein powder, unflavored
4 oz salted caramel Greek yogurt, fat-free
1 egg

8 oz Greek yogurt cream cheese, low-fat and softened

Instructions

Crust:

Your oven should be at 325.

Place parchment into the bottom of four mini spring form pans.

Pulse up the cream cheese and the cereal until it becomes clumpy. Press the crust into each of the pans and bake them for about ten minutes.

Cheesecake:

Beat together the sweetener, protein powder, vanilla, yogurt, egg, and cream cheese. Beat at medium speed for a minute and then increase it to high for another two minutes. Make sure all of the lumps have been removed.

Place the cream cheese over the crust. Put the pans into a casserole dish. Put boiling water into a separate baking dish a sit it on the bottom rack of your oven. Put the dish of cheesecakes on the middle rack. Let this bake for 30 minutes.

Switch your oven off and slightly crack your oven door. Let them stay there until the cool.

Carefully release the spring form pan and slide the cheesecake off by the parchment paper.

Mini Strawberry Cheesecakes

Ingredients

Crust:

1 tbsp sugar

¼ c butter, melted

1 c graham cracker crumbs

Filling:

5 drops red food coloring

2 5oz containers Greek yogurt, strawberry

2 eggs

¼ tsp salt

½ c strawberry jams

2/3 c sugar

1 tbsp cornstarch

1 tsp vanilla

2 8oz pack 1/3 fat cream cheese

Topping:

15 strawberries

1 c whipped cream, fat-free

Instructions

Crust:

Your oven should be at 325. Put liners into a regular muffin tin.

Mix together the sugar, butter, and graham crackers. Press a tablespoon of this into every one of the cupcakes tins

Filling:

Beat together the sugar, salt, cornstarch, and creams cheese until it becomes fluffy. Mix in the food coloring, vanilla, and strawberry jam. Make sure it is mixed well. Mix an egg one at a time. Stir in the Greek yogurt.

Pour the mixture into the cups over the crusts. The liners should be filled almost all the way to the top. Cook for 20 to 22 minutes. The edges should be set with the centers wobbly

Let them cool for 30 minutes. Set them out on a wire rack and allow them to completely cool. Place in the fridge for at least four hours before you serve them.

Top the cheese cake with whipped cream and strawberries.

Blueberry Cookies

Ingredients

2 scoops vanilla protein powder

1 c berries

½ c oatmeal

4 egg whites

Instructions

Stir the oatmeal, egg whites, and protein powder together until well combined.

Mix in the berries of your choice.

Drop spoonfuls of you cookie dough onto a nonstick coated cookie sheet.

Your oven should be at 425. Bake them for 10 to 15 minutes.

Strawberry Cheesecake

Ingredients

4 tsp Splenda

2 c strawberries, halved

½ fat-free cool whip

1 c nonfat milk

½ pkg sugar-free cheesecake pudding

4 oz. fat-free ricotta cheese

Instructions

Wash strawberries and cut them in half. Add Splenda and gently mix. Set to the side.

Add milk, pudding mix, and ricotta to blender. Blend until creamy and smooth. Pour into a bowl but not with the strawberries. Add cool whip and gently fold.

Spoon a small amount of the pudding mix into serving dishes. Add strawberries. Continue layering there you have used up all ingredients. Top with any remaining strawberries.

Pumpkin Pie Cheesecake

Ingredients

¼ tsp ground allspice

4 egg whites

½ tsp ground cinnamon

1 c canned pumpkin

¼ tsp ground nutmeg

1 c sugar substitute

3 8 oz. pkg fat-free cream cheese

1 tsp vanilla extract

Instructions

Heat oven to 375.

Blend vanilla, sugar, and cream cheese together in a bowl with electric mixer. Add spices, eggs, and pumpkin. Blend until it is smooth.

Pour into a 9-inch spring form pan. You can use a pie crust if wanted.

Bake between 60 and 70 minutes until top turns lightly brown. Remove and cool to room temp

Refrigerate until it is chilled.

Once chilled, remove from spring form pan and cut.

Serve with the fat-free cool whip or whipped cream.

Apple Cake

Ingredients

¼ c chopped walnuts

1 tsp cinnamon

1 c all-purpose flour

½ tsp salt

½ tsp baking powder

4 tbsp butter

4 medium diced apples

½ tsp baking soda

½ tsp nutmeg

1 c Splenda

1 egg

Instructions

Heat oven to 350.

Peel, core, and dice the apples.

Grease an 8-inch square pan.

Blend butter and sugar together.

Beat egg, add walnuts and vanilla. Combine. Add to apples. Add butter mixture and mix it together.

Sift remaining ingredients and add to apple mixture. Mix well. Pour into prepared pan. Cook about 45 minutes. Allow it to cool and then cut into squares.

Fruit Dip

Ingredients

6 oz. fat-free, sugar-free vanilla yogurt

8 oz. low-fat cream cheese, softened

3 tbsp. Splenda

1 tsp vanilla

Instructions

Beat up the cream cheese. Add Splenda, vanilla, and yogurt slowly. Increase speed and blend until fluffy and light.

Use as a dip for favorite fruit.

Mousse

Ingredients

2 c boiling water

3 scoops vanilla protein powder

2 small boxes sugar free jello favorite flavor

24 oz 1% cottage cheese

Instructions

Boil two cups water. Add jello and stir until dissolved. Let cool a few minutes.

But cottage cheese into a blender. Blend out the lumps.

Mix in cooled jello and protein powder. Blend until well mixed.

Divide into six serving dishes. Chill overnight. This will have a very light mousse-like consistency.

Serve and enjoy.

Cheesecake Pudding

Ingredients

1 cup plain fat-free Greek yogurt

1 pkg sugar-free cheesecake pudding mix

Instructions

Mix all of the above ingredients together.

I Can't Believe It's Not Cheesecake

Ingredients

1 small pkg sugar-free flavored gelatin, your choice of flavor

2 tbsp. Splenda

2 8 oz. pkg low-fat cream cheese

1 cup boiling water

1 6 oz container Greek yogurt, plain

Instructions

Mix water and gelatin until dissolved. Add cream cheese and yogurt. Mix with electric mixer until thoroughly combined. Taste. Add Splenda if needed.

Put in fridge overnight.

Once ready to serve, garnish with fruit, sugar-free cookie crumbs, or whipped cream.

Strawberry Dessert

Ingredients

4 c fresh sliced strawberries

2 8 oz tubs light cool whip

2 small boxes sugar-free strawberry jello

32 oz container 4% cottage cheese

Instructions

Combine jello mix and cottage cheese. Combine. Mix in the cool whip and strawberries. Chill.

Pumpkin Protein Pie

Ingredients

2 scoops unflavored whey protein

2 oz. pkg pecan halves

1 tsp nutmeg

½ tsp salt

1/3 cup Splenda

1 tsp cinnamon

1 c ricotta cheese, low-fat

1 c nonfat milk

2 large eggs

2 c pumpkin puree

Instructions

Heat oven to 350. Spray 4 small ramekins and 9-inch pie plate with cooking spray.

Blend ½ cup milk, eggs, and ricotta cheese until smooth. It will be liquid.

Add all the rest and mix up again.

Place into sprayed cooking dishes. Place pecans on top.

Bake 45 minutes or until middle is almost solid. There should be no jiggle if cooked through. The center and sides will brown and grow to double the size. If yours starts to burn, reduce temperature to 325 for rest of cooking time.

Take it out from the oven and allow it to cool for one hour before you cut. Slice it into 12 equal pieces. Wipe between cuts.

Silky Chocolate Dessert

Ingredients

¼ tsp peppermint extract

1 pkg sugar-free chocolate fudge instant pudding

1 tbsp cocoa powder

½ tsp vanilla extract

16 oz silken tofu

1 c skim milk

¼ c hot water

1 envelope unflavored gelatin

Instructions

Mix unflavored gelatin and hot water in small bowl. Set aside and let firm.

Combine instant pudding mix and milk in another bowl. Dice tofu into cubes and put in a bowl alongside of the pudding. Whisk vigorously to break up soy cubes. Add peppermint extract, cocoa powder, and vanilla.

Spoon into a blender. Blend smooth. You might have to shake the blender, so ingredients don't stick. When the mixture has reached a smoothie consistency, add gelatin until combined. Blend one more time.

Pour into 8-inch glass pie plate. Cover and put in the fridge for about 30 minutes to get firm. Cut into eight equal pieces and enjoy.

Snacks and Appetizers

Potato and Crab Salad

Ingredients

Lemon wedge

Smoked salmon and green salad – optional

Pepper

Salt

4 tbsp snipped chives

½ lemon, juiced

2 tbsp Greek yogurt, fat-free

2 tbsp mayonnaise, extra light

6 oz cooked crab meat

8 medium potatoes, cooked

Instructions

Dice up the potatoes up and put them in a bowl with your flaked crab meat.

Mix together the pepper, chives, salt, lemon juice, yogurt, and mayonnaise. Adjust the pepper and salt as you need to.

Place the mixed dressing over the crab and potatoes and toss together, so it's all well coated.

Serve this with some smoked salmon and a green salad along with a lemon wedge for a complete meal.

Blackberry and Chicken Salad

Ingredients

2 sprigs thyme, chopped

½ to 1 tsp honey

½ lemon, zest

2 tbsp vinaigrette dressing, fat-free or low-fat

1 c blackberries

2 oz feta cheese, light

1 bunch watercress, trimmed

1 cooked chicken breast, shredded

2 tsp olive oil

2 slices walnut bread, chunked

Instructions

Your oven should be at 400. Place the bread onto a cookie sheet and top with oil. Bake these for about five minutes or until the crisp up.

Put the blackberries, feta, watercress, and chicken in a bowl. Top with the fresh croutons.

Combine the thyme, honey, lemon, and vinaigrette and stir well. Place the mixture on top of the salad and toss everything together.

Caprese Salad

Ingredients

Pepper

Salt

2 to 3 tbsp balsamic dressing

Handful salad leaves

7 oz mozzarella, light and sliced

1 ripe avocado, scoop into balls – dip them in lemon juice to keep from oxidizing

6 oz strawberries, sliced

Instructions

Mix together the salad leaves, mozzarella, avocado, and strawberries

Drizzle the balsamic dressing over the top and add a generous amount of pepper and salt.

Toss everything together and enjoy.

Grape Salad

Ingredients

½ c chopped walnuts or pecans

¼ c brown sugar

4 tsp vanilla extract

½ c Splenda

8 oz. fat-free sour cream

2 to 4 lbs red or green grapes

Instructions

Wash and dry grapes. Put grapes in large bowl. Using a hand mixer, blend vanilla, Splenda, sour cream, and cream cheese until mixed well.

Fold into grapes until well coated. Put in 9 X 13 cake pan. Top with the brown sugar and chopped nuts.

Put in refrigerator for an hour.

Chicken Salad

Ingredients

3 tbsp miracle whip light

½ c quartered grapes

¼ c craisins

¼ c diced celery

1 ½ c diced, grilled chicken breast

Instructions

Place all ingredients in a bowl. May be served over a bed of greens or as a sandwich.

Corn and Black Bean Salad

Ingredients

¼ tsp black pepper

1 tsp honey

2 tbsp olive oil

1 tsp lemon juice

¼ c balsamic vinegar

Salt

2 cans 16 oz black beans, drained and rinsed

2 tbsp minced red onion

¼ c chopped fresh parsley

1 tsp minced garlic

1 c whole kernel corn

Instructions

Mix parsley, onion, black beans, and corn together in large bowl.

Whisk pepper, salt, honey, garlic, lemon juice, olive oil, balsamic vinegar together.

Pour over corn and black beans. Stir to coat.

Let stand for 30 minutes.

Serve over a bed of lettuce, with pita chips, or tortilla chips.

Aunt Faye's Chicken Salad

Ingredients

¼ c sliced almonds

1 c red seedless grapes, halved

1 c light sour cream

¼ c light miracle whip

½ tsp celery seed

3 tbsp lemon juice

3 lb cooked, cubed chicken breast

Instructions

Put chicken in large bowl. Add lemon juice, celery seed, sour cream, miracle whip. Stir well. Add almonds and grapes. Give another stir. Place in refrigerator for one hour.

Serve with crackers or flour tortillas.

Grape and Chicken Salad

Ingredients

¼ c walnuts

2 tbsp light mayonnaise

1 c sliced grapes

1 lb grilled chicken

Instructions

Mix everything up in a bowl. Place on a sandwich or lettuce bed.

Baked Zucchini

Ingredients

1 oz 1% milk

1 large egg white

½ c Italian bread crumbs

2 tbsp grated parmesan

2 c sliced zucchini

Instructions

Your oven should be at 400. Spray the baking sheet with nonstick spray.

Combine the dry ingredients in shallow dish.

Stir the milk and egg whites together in a different shallow dish.

Place zucchini slices in milk mixture. Cover with bread crumbs.

Lay in one layer on baking sheet. Spritz with oil spray.

Fry for ten minutes and then flip them over. Fry for another ten minutes until it has crisped up and browned

Salmon Cakes

Ingredients

Salt

1 tsp garlic powder

1 large egg

1 tsp pepper

1 can salmon

1 c diced onion

Instructions

Check salmon for bones and remove. This step gets messy.

Combine everything and make them into patty shapes. Fry like you would a hamburger.

Serve like a hamburger or over a bed of greens.

Standard Chicken Salad

Ingredients

Salt

Pepper

Pinch cayenne

Pinch curry powder

1 tsp mustard

3 tbsp light mayonnaise

1 ½ c chopped celery

1 ½ c cooked, chopped chicken

Instructions

Mix all ingredients well. Season to taste. Place on a lettuce bed.

Deviled Eggs

Ingredients

1 tsp pepper

2 cloves crushed garlic

1 tsp salt

1 tsp onion powder

3 tbsp. fat-free mayonnaise

3 tbsp. Dijon mustard

6 hard-boiled eggs

Instructions

Slice in half long way. Gently take out the yolks and place in a bowl. Use a fork and mash the yolks until fine. Add remaining ingredients. Mix well. Using spoon, place yolk mixture into egg whites.

Hummus

Ingredients

¼ tsp salt

1 tsp chopped garlic

¾ c plain nonfat yogurt

1 16 oz can chickpeas or garbanzo beans

1 ½ tbsp. lemon juice

Instructions

Drain and rinse beans. Put this stuff in your food processor. Mix up until creamy and smooth

Taste test and adjust seasoning if needed. Add cilantro, red pepper, and cumin if desired.

Serve with pita chips or tortilla chips.

Cucumber Soup

Ingredients

1 medium seeded and diced tomato

Salt

Pepper

3 tbsp chopped dill

1 scallion chopped include green parts

1 English cucumber, chunked

2 tsp olive oil

3 cups plain nonfat yogurt

Instructions

Combine dill, scallion, cucumber, and yogurt in a blender. Pulse until smooth. Taste and season accordingly. Ladle into bowls. Top with diced tomato, a drizzle of olive oil and dill sprig.

Serve with a piece of whole grain bread.

Tuna Patties

Ingredients

1 tbsp parmesan cheese

Dash garlic powder

1 large egg

Dash onion powder

1 tbsp light mayonnaise

2 tbsp flax meal

1 pouch tuna in water

Instructions

Drain tuna. Mash with a fork to make smaller. Mix all ingredients with a fork. Form into four patties. Fry in sauté pan greased with nonstick spray until it has browned.

Black Bean Salad

Ingredients

3 cloves garlic, minced

1 tbsp diced cilantro

1 onion, chopped

1 tsp cumin

1 can whole kernel corn, drained

¼ cup apple cider vinegar

1 tsp cayenne pepper

1 tbsp olive oil

1 red bell pepper, chopped and seed removed

¼ cup water

1 can black beans, washed and drained

Instructions

Sauté the onion and the bell pepper together in the oil until they become soft. Mix in garlic, cook until it smells. Add cayenne, cumin, cilantro, corn, vinegar, water, and black beans. Let it come to a boil. Turn it to simmer. When the mixture has reduced slightly, it is ready to eat.

Serve with pita or tortilla chips.

Tuna and Apple Sandwich

Ingredients

3 lettuce leaves

6 slices whole wheat bread

½ tsp honey

1 tsp mustard

¼ c low-fat vanilla yogurt

1 apple

1 can tuna, packed in water, drained

Instructions

Wash the apple. Peel, core, and chop. Put the apple in a bowl. Add tuna, honey, mustard, and yogurt. Stir well. Spread ½ cup onto three slices of bread. Top with lettuce leaves and the other slice of bread.

Chicken Cheesesteak Wrap

Ingredients

2 tsp sliced pickled hot chili peppers

1 whole wheat flour tortilla

¼ lb boneless skinless chicken breast

1 wedge swiss cheese spread

½ c sliced mushrooms

¼ c sliced green pepper

¼ c chopped onion

Instructions

Put chicken on cutting board and pound to ¼-inch thickness. Slice into strips. Spray the skillet with a nonstick cooking spray, or you can brush it with a very little amount of oil as an alternative.

Place the onion and the chicken cooking until the chicken is done. Mix in mushrooms and green peppers. Cook until mushrooms and pepper are soft.

Put tortilla between two damp paper towels. Microwave 20 seconds.

Put tortilla on a plate and put Swiss cheese in a strip down the middle. Top with mushrooms, onions, peppers, and chicken. Add pickled chili peppers. Fold sides over the middle. Serve and enjoy.

Faux Fried Rice

Ingredients

Olive oil spray
2 large egg whites
1 tsp chili paste
¼ c frozen peas
¾ c cooked brown rice
1 clove minced garlic
1 tsp mustard
¼ c chopped carrot
½ c finely chopped green onions
2 tbsp low sodium soy sauce
Pepper
3 oz boneless, skinless chicken breast, cubed

1 tsp toasted sesame oil

Instructions

Combine sesame oil, chili paste, mustard, and soy sauce in small bowl. Set to the side for later use.

Place pepper on chicken. Coat a pan with nonstick spray. Once heated, place chicken in skillet.

Cook all the way through so that it is no longer pink.

Keep the chicken warm.

Spray skillet again with nonstick spray. Add garlic, carrot, and green onions. Cook a few minutes. Add peas and rice. Cook for two minutes so that everything is heated.

Create a hole in the center of rice. Lightly spray exposed part with cooking spray. Add egg whites. Stir to mix into rice. Cook until egg is cooked through.

Put chicken back into the pan. Stir well. Add soy sauce mixture. Continue to cook constantly stirring until heated.

Serve and enjoy.

Ranch Style Salad

Ingredients

2 tbsp garlic and herb soft cheese, light

4 oz bag baby leaf herb salad

1 romaine lettuce head, torn roughly

3 tbsp white wine vinegar

¾ c hard cheese, grated and low-fat

1 red pepper, chopped and seeded

14 oz. kidney beans, washed and drained

11 oz sweet corn

Low-fat spray

Instructions

Spray a generous amount of low-fat spray on your skillet and let it heat up. Add in the sweet corn and let it cook until charred a little.

Combine the cheese, red pepper, and kidney beans together. Stir in the salad leaves and the lettuce.

For the dressing combine three tablespoons of water, the vinegar, and the soft cheese. Add the corn and then drizzle on the dressing. Toss everything together.

Zucchini Chips

Ingredients

Salt

Pepper

1 tbsp parsley, chopped

3 tbsp parmesan, grated

Nonstick spray

3 zucchini, sliced into chips

Instructions

Your oven should be at 425. Place parchment paper onto a rimmed cookie sheet. Put the zucchini slices on the cookie sheet and spray them with some non-stick spray. Combine the salt, parsley, pepper, and parmesan together. Sprinkle this over the zucchini chips. Bake this until the cheese melts, and the zucchini has crisped up but hasn't burned. This should take about 30 minutes.

Mozzarella Sticks

Ingredients

1 tsp olive oil

½ c marinara sauce – dipping

8 wonton wrappers

4 string cheese sticks, halved

1 egg

Instructions

In a bowl, mix together a tablespoon of water and the egg. One at a time, brush each of the wrappers with the egg wash.

Put a string cheese half in the middle of each one of the wrappers; there should be a corner at each end and top and bottom of the wrapper. Take the bottom corner and fold it over the cheese. Bring the two side corners in, and then roll the cheese stick up to the top corner. Make sure you are careful and don't tear the wrappers.

Add some of the olive oil into your skillet and let heat. Place the mozzarella sticks and cook them until they are golden.

Serve with the marinara sauce.

Ranch Cauliflower Bites

Ingredients

1 tsp chives

6 bacon strips, cooked and crumbled

1 ¼ cheddar cheese, shredded and divided

1 ranch seasoning packet

2 egg

1 cauliflower head

Instructions

Your oven should be at 375.

Place the cauliflower in your food processor and pulse it up until it becomes large crumbs.

Put the cauliflower crumbs on a cheesecloth or paper towels and wring out any excess water. Place the drained cauliflower into a bowl.

Add in the chives, ¾ s of the bacon, ranch seasoning, one cup of cheese, and the eggs.

Spray a regular muffin tin with nonstick spray and then fill them up to 2/3s full. Sprinkle the top with bacon and cheese. Place them in the oven for around 20 to 22 minutes. They will turn golden. Top with additional chives if desired.

Peanut Butter Roll-Up

Ingredients

½ tbsp honey

½ banana

1 tbsp peanut butter

1 flatbread

Instructions

Spread your peanut butter over you flatbread. Slice up the banana and place them over the flatbread on top of the peanut butter. Drizzle the honey over everything. Roll it up, slice in half, and then enjoy.

Extras

Blueberry and Basil Water

Ingredients

1-pint blueberries

Bunch of basil

Pitcher of water

Instructions

Rinse blueberries and basil. Crush blueberries and place in the water pitcher. Leave basil on stems and add to pitcher. Fill with water. Refrigerate for a few hours. When you let it sit for a while, it will taste better. You can just keep adding water to the fruit.

Mint and Cucumber Water

Ingredients

3 English cucumber

1 bunch mint

Pitcher of water

Instructions

Rinse cucumber and mint. Thinly slice the cucumbers and place in pitcher. The more cucumbers, the more the water will be flavored. Leave mint on stems add to pitcher. Fill with water. Refrigerate for a few hours. The longer it sits, the better the flavor. You can keep adding water to the pitcher for more flavored water.

Watermelon Water

Ingredients

1 small watermelon

Pitcher of water

Instructions

Cube watermelon and put in pitcher. The more watermelon, the faster the water will be flavored. You may add mint if you prefer. Let sit for several hours. If you let it sit for a while, it will taste better. You can reuse the fruit by adding more water to the pitcher.

Sugar-free Lemonade with Strawberries

Ingredients

1-quart strawberries

1 lemon thinly sliced

Pitcher of water

Instructions

Rinse strawberries. Grate strawberries into a pitcher. Add lemons. Let sit several hours in the refrigerator. The longer it sits, the better the taste. The fruit can be reused by adding more water.

Infused Ice Cubes

Ingredients

Ice cube tray

Boiling water

Herbs and fruits of choice

Instructions

Add any chopped fruit or herbs to ice cube tray. Pour boiling water over. Let cool before you place it in the freezer. When you heat the fruits and herbs, you release their flavor. This gives the ice cube flavor.

Peanut Salad Dressing

Ingredients

1/8 tsp garlic powder

1 tbsp. water

1 tsp Splenda brown sugar

¼ tsp Szechuan chili sauce

1 tbsp. low sodium soy sauce

¼ tsp ground pepper

1/8 tsp sesame oil

2 tbsp. powdered peanuts

Instructions

Put the above in a blender and mix well. Refrigerate any leftovers.

Conclusion

Thank for making it through to the end of *Gastric Bypass Cookbook*. Let's hope it was informative and able to provide you with all of the tools you need to achieve your goals.

The next step is to use these books to make sure that you have success after your gastric bypass surgery.

Finally, if you found this book useful in any way, a review on Amazon is always appreciated!

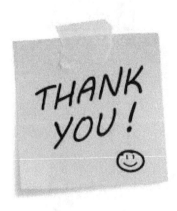

Check Out My Other Books

Below you'll find some of my other popular books that are popular on Amazon and Kindle as well. Simply click on the links below to check them out. Alternatively, you can visit my author page on Amazon to see other work done by me.

CrossFit: Barbell and Dumbbell Exercises for Body Strength

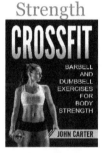

Mediterranean Diet: Step By Step Guide And Proven Recipes For Smart Eating And Weight Loss

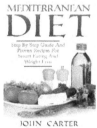

Weight Watchers:
Smart Points Cookbook - Step By Step Guide And
Proven Recipes For Effective Weight Loss

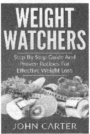

Bodybuilding: Beginners Handbook - Proven Step By
Step Guide To Get The Body You Always Dreamed
About

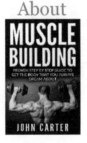

South Beach Diet: Lose Weight and Get Healthy the
South Beach Way

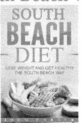

Blood Pressure: Step By Step Guide And Proven
Recipes To Lower Your Blood Pressure Without Any
Medication

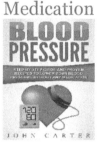

Ketogenic Diet: Step By Step Guide And 70+ Low
Carb, Proven Recipes For Rapid Weight Loss

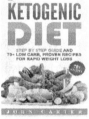

Meal Prep: 65+ Meal Prep Recipes Cookbook – Step
By Step Meal Prepping Guide For Rapid Weight Loss

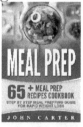

If the links do not work, for whatever reason, you can
simply search for these titles on the Amazon website to
find them.